Allergies

ALLERGIES
by Sarah R. Riedman

◄ A FIRST BOOK ►

FRANKLIN WATTS | NEW YORK | LONDON | 1978

Cover design by Ginger Giles

Photographs courtesy of:
Allergy Foundation of America: pp. 5, 14 (top right); Dr. Earl B. Brown: p. 14 (top left); Dr. Frank Perlman/C.D.C.: pp. 14 (bottom), 43; Sterling Drug Inc./Breon Laboratories: pp. 20, 33; Schering Corporation: p. 38; Medic Alert Foundation: p. 46; Center for Disease Control: p. 49; Greer Laboratories, Inc.: 52.

Library of Congress Cataloging in Publication Data

Riedman, Sarah R
    Allergies.

    (A First book)
    Bibliography: p.
    Includes index.
    SUMMARY: Describes the symptoms, causes, and treatment of allergies including food allergies, hay fever, asthma, and insect stings.
    1. Allergy—Juvenile literature. [1. Allergy] I. Title.
RC584.R53   616.9'7   77-20858
ISBN 0-531-01352-9

Copyright © 1978 by Sarah R. Riedman
All rights reserved
Printed in the United States of America
6 5 4 3 2 1

Contents

1
SO, YOU'RE ALLERGIC
1

2
THE STRANGE ALLERGEN
IN THIS CASE
9

3
ALL CLUES LEAD
TO ALLERGIC RHINITIS
17

4
HAY FEVER
24

5
ASTHMA
29

6
WHEN FOOD IS THE ALLERGEN
35

7
DON'T LET A BEE STING AGAIN
41

8
IS IT SOMETHING YOU TOUCHED?
48

GLOSSARY
56

FURTHER READING
60

INDEX
62

Allergies

1

So, You're Allergic

Michael came to school with a runny nose. Throughout the day he kept rubbing his nose as if it were itchy. The teacher told him to tell his mother to keep him home until his nose stopped running. Or else other children would catch his cold. The next day Michael's mother sent him to school with a note from his doctor. It read: "Michael's condition is not the common cold, but PERENNIAL ALLERGIC RHINITIS." RHINITIS means an irritated lining of the nose. In Michael's case it was due to a HYPERSENSITIVITY. This meant that he was sensitive to a certain food, a pet's fur, or some plant, making him sick. His was not an infection, like a cold, but an ALLERGY. And it was not contagious (catching).

    Allergies and infections have one thing in common: both are caused by something foreign entering the body. The body recognizes it as foreign and has ways of attacking it. The way the body defends itself is called its REACTION. But in many other ways, allergies and infections differ.

TWO KINDS OF INVADERS

In an infection the "invader" is a living thing: a virus, a bacterium (plural: bacteria), or a fungus (mold is an example).

Colds and influenza (flu), measles and mumps are caused by viruses. Scarlet fever and whooping cough are caused by bacteria. And ringworm is caused—not by a worm—by a fungus. These are all living parasites. But an allergy is due to a chemical, usually a protein (the most important chemical of living cells), or some other complex substance in a food or in the air. The strange thing is that the substance makes only *some* people sick. We say these people are allergic to that substance. It could be as common a food as an egg, or as ordinary a plant as grass. Anyone can get measles, but only *certain people* are allergic to egg-white protein or to cat fur.

What causes Michael's allergy may be hard to track down. But someone else in his family may also be allergic, although not necessarily to the same thing, and may show it in a different way. That it runs in the family is one clue the doctor will follow up, as we will see later.

TWO WAYS TO STRIKE BACK

In an infection the disease starter is the ANTIGEN. In an allergy, the foreign chemical is the ALLERGEN. Both trigger the body to manufacture products to act against each special antigen and allergen. These are called ANTIBODIES, the body's defense chemicals made by certain cells, which then circulate in the blood. Each antibody links up with its special antigen or allergen, fitting it like a lock and key, so as to block its harmful action.

SICK EITHER WAY—
BUT WITH A DIFFERENCE

A child with measles is very sick for at least a few days. First a high fever, a temperature up to 104°F. (40°C.) develops (98.6°F. [37°C.] is normal). Then a rash breaks out on the face and behind the ears, spreading to the neck and chest. The throat is sore, the nose runs, and the eyes are red and sensitive to light. The infection jogs the body into making antibodies, and steadily the child gets better. The fever goes down, the rash fades, and the other symptoms (signs of disease) disappear. The wonder is that the built-up antibodies remain in the blood for life. They ward off another attack, and we say the person is now IMMUNE to measles. Measles is highly contagious for anyone who has not had it.

How very different with allergies! As Michael's doctor wrote, his allergy is not catching. He did not catch it from anyone, nor can he spread it to anyone else. Michael is probably allergic to something in the air, although it doesn't bother anyone else in his home or outdoors. Very likely he did not show the allergic signs until he was four or five years old. Just what started it? It could be so many different things that give him his reaction that it may take an ALLERGIST (a doctor—"detective") to find out. An allergy could also show up only days or weeks after a baby is born. If it happens that early, a food is suspected, perhaps milk, or orange juice, or a cereal, as solid food is added to the baby's diet.

AN ALLERGY FOR LIFE

Unless the cause of Michael's allergy is discovered, he will get repeated attacks. They will occur more often and each attack may well be worse. If the cause is known, he can be treated so that his attacks will be less severe and less frequent. But he will not become altogether immune. He will not outgrow his allergy.

What about those antibodies that his body produces against his special allergen? Here lies the big difference between the way the body reacts to an allergen and the way it reacts to a measles or chicken pox virus.

The first time the allergen entered his body, it may not have produced any visible signs. But something did happen in his body. We say Michael became SENSITIZED. This means that the second time he was exposed to or came in contact with that allergen, he had an attack. Oddly enough, it was his antibodies that brought on his sneezing, made his nose run, and his eyes and nose itchy. The reason? The linking up of allergen and antibody starts off a process that releases a number of damaging chemicals, among them one called HISTAMINE.

It is as if the body overreacted and the defenses were overpowered. In fact, the word "allergy" comes from two Greek words, *allos,* meaning "other" and *ergon,* meaning "work."

So we see that allergies tend to run in families, are not contagious, and don't usually start up a fever. Their cause is hard to pinpoint, and the antibodies do not make the person immune. Allergies are not cured the way infections can be. But the symptoms may be relieved, the chance of later attacks lessened, and the discomfort weakened by the right treatment.

Four common allergens—ragweed, Bermuda grass, sagebrush and English plantain—with their American distribution and pollen samples.

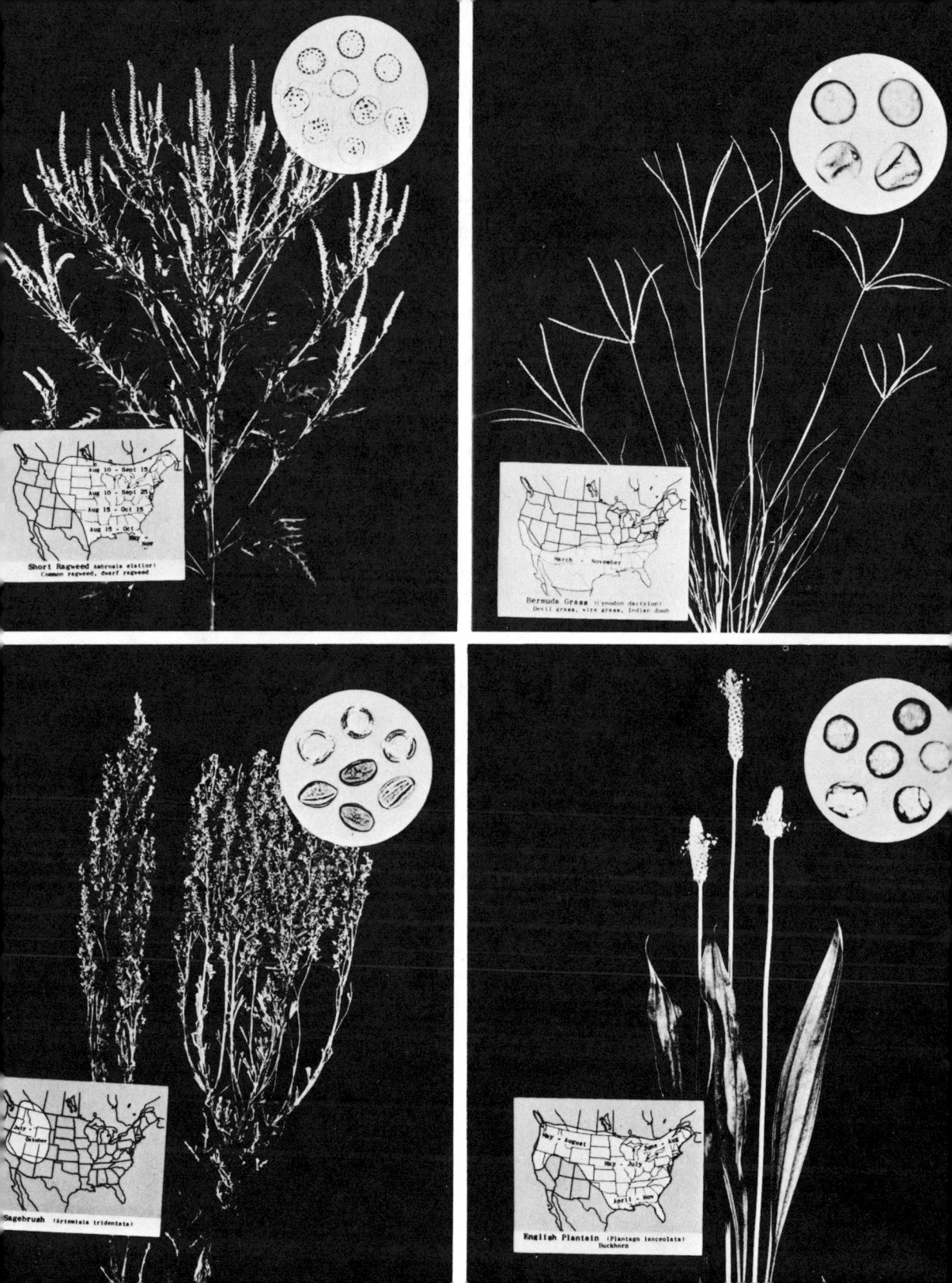

ALLERGENS BY THE HUNDREDS

The number of possible allergens seems countless. Let's look at a shortened list, grouped by kinds.

1. INHALANTS (substances breathed in):

POLLEN (fine powdery stuff from the male part of a flower); mold SPORES ("seeds" of fungi); animal DANDER (tiny scales from hair, fur, and feathers) of horses, rabbits, cats, dogs, birds; house dust; cotton lint and bits of other textile fibers; cottonseed pressed for oil, made into fertilizer meal, and animal feed; yarns, jute (for twine, rope, carpets); wool in hats, rugs, blankets.

(You might say that Michael had little or no chance to handle or be near most of these things. But he could have played with a toy stuffed with cat fur, or taken a pony ride—horsehair, you see.)

Other inhalants may be even harder to track down. One insecticide, pyrethrum, used on farms or against household insect pests is made from a plant from the same family as dandelions, asters, goldenrods—and ragweed! Ragweed has a bad reputation as an allergen. Even food odors, from an opened can of sardines, or fish being cooked, can bring on a rash or make breathing difficult for someone sensitized to fish.

2. INGESTANTS (anything taken in by mouth):

FOODS. The most common allergenic foods are milk, eggs, cereals, particularly wheat; fish, nuts, chocolate, spices (mustard seed is one); less often fruits, but strawberries, bananas, oranges, and peaches are on the allergenic list. This means custard, puddings, or cakes made with milk; bread, cookies, noodles made from wheat flour; and strawberry pie. Foods and drinks to which a food coloring is added; syrups, candies, popsicles, bubble gum, and soda pop also belong on the list.

DRUGS. Penicillin is one drug to which some people are sensitive and can get a violent reaction to. A baby nursed by its mother may become allergic through the mother's milk, if she has taken penicillin. Aspirin is another drug on the forbidden list of some allergic persons.

3. INJECTABLES:

It does not matter how an allergen is introduced into the body. For example, penicillin, whether swallowed as a capsule or syrup, or injected, can cause a reaction. Or a vaccine prepared from a chick embryo in the egg will produce a reaction when vaccinating a child allergic to eggs. Introduced into the body in an enema or suppository, a drug may also arouse a reaction in someone sensitive to that drug.

4. CHEMICALS JUST TOUCHED:

Just touching or coming in contact with certain plants or chemicals may cause a rash and itching. Poison ivy doesn't have to be eaten, but touching the plant, or handling newsprint ink, certain dyes, paints and turpentine may cause a *contact* reaction.

ALLERGY SIGNS AND WHERE THEY SHOW

Rashes, blebs or welts, wheals (white raised spots on the skin), sneezing, wheezing, dry rasping cough, troubled breathing, snoring, watery stream from the nose, and tearing eyes that itch or smart are some allergy symptoms. So also may be vomiting, nausea, DIARRHEA (loose and frequent bowel movements), and cramps; also some kinds of headache may be due to a foreign chemical.

From these symptoms you can figure out where the signs show: on the skin, eyes, nose, lungs; in the stomach and intestines, and in the small blood vessels. These are called the *target* or *shock* organs.

Michael's allergy showed up in his nose and eyes—the shock organs in his case. The name his doctor gave it was only one kind of allergy. For other allergies—how they are named, how the causes are searched for, what methods are used, and how the allergic patient is treated—read on.

2

The Strange Allergen in this Case

Andrew Jones, a fire fighter, quite suddenly developed a dry, hacking cough, had pain in his chest, trouble breathing, and at times was feverish during the hours he was in the firehouse. He was accustomed to choking on smoke on entering a burning building, but why in the firehouse? Neither on the fire truck rushing to the scene of a fire, nor at home did he have this troublesome, choked-up feeling.

The doctor looked at his throat, examined the inside of his nose, listened to his chest. Since the patient complained of his severe discomfort only while on duty at the firehouse, the doctor suspected an allergy. An allergist was needed in order to detect the cause, if indeed it was an allergy.

Allergists usually begin by asking their patient to fill in a lengthy questionnaire. The answers help track down a number of likely clues. Some answers to the questions may lead to a dead end. Still they are helpful in telling which direction *not* to follow for further clues.

A HEAP OF QUESTIONS

An allergist's questionnaire could look something like this:

1. What are your complaints? Check which: Itching ☐ Sneezing ☐ Watering eyes ☐ Difficult breathing ☐ Headache ☐ Others ☐

2. When did you first have any of these symptoms? Where and under what circumstances? Explain in your own words.

3. Do you feel worse when exposed to cold air ☐ dampness ☐ strong wind? ☐

4. Are the symptoms worse out of doors, in the house, at work, in public places: church, crowded buses, subways? ☐

5. Do certain fumes, odors of fresh paint, or smoke bring on your symptoms? ☐

6. What foods, if any, disagree with you, give nausea, cause burping, vomiting, abdominal cramps?

7. Does anyone in your family have similar symptoms? ☐

8. Do any of them have asthma, hay fever, allergic bronchitis? ☐

9. Do some kinds of fabrics make you itch? Give you a rash? Wool ☐ silk ☐

10. Do you have pets? A cat ☐ dog ☐ a parakeet? ☐

11. Do you have contact with horses? ☐ farm animals? ☐

/10/

12. Have you recently been ill? ☐ With what? ☐

13. Did you take any drug that you have never had before? ☐

14. Did you ever have a bad reaction to a vaccination or a tetanus shot ☐ flu vaccine ☐ penicillin or any other drug? ☐

15. Has there been any change in the furnishings of your home? ☐ new upholstery, carpet, or hangings? ☐

In the case of Mr. Jones, practically all of the possible clues could be ruled out. He could answer "no" to most of the questions. There was no known family history of allergy. He always had a dog, and as far as he knew nothing had changed in home surroundings or at his place of work. The only suspicious clue was the discomfort and labored breathing in the firehouse.

LOOKING YOU OVER

Next came the physical examination. The doctor took note of Mr. Jones's dry cough. Usually, with an infection, sputum sometimes with pus accompanies the cough. The doctor had Mr. Jones breathe through a tube into an instrument that measures the volume of air breathed out after taking the deepest possible breath. Yes, the patient had less than the normal breathing capacity for a man in otherwise good health. Listening to Mr. Jones's lungs the doctor heard an abnormal sound. The doctor wrote down *rales,* the French word for "rattle." Next, a chest X ray was taken. Mostly the lungs were clear, except for a speckling and blotching of cell groups in the lower part of the lungs. The doctor had a name for this disease, commonly called "farmers' lung," "pigeon breeders' lung," or "maple-bark strippers' disease." In farmers' lung, the allergen is in moldy hay. Pigeon raisers get it from exposure to the birds' feathers and droppings, and in maple-bark strippers' disease the allergen is a mold.

But why would a fire fighter have an allergic condition that was linked to pigeons, parakeets, or molds on hay? Could it be that some bird or other animal was seeking refuge in the firehouse? The answer was not in the questionnaire, but it suddenly hit Mr. Jones that one of the fire fighters was looking after a pair of caged *gerbils* left in his care by a vacationing relative. That could be it! The gerbils had to go, at least to see if Mr. Jones would be freed of his trouble. Yes, the fire fighter's uneasy breathing was relieved, but the allergist needed the final proof, by a test. An injection of a highly watered down bit of gerbil dander in the patient's skin brought on the difficult breathing for Mr. Jones. What's more, his blood contained the antibody against the gerbil antigen. If any further proof was needed, it came months later when Mr. Jones choked up again while visiting the home where the gerbils had once been housed, but were removed just before the fire fighter's visit. The traces of gerbil dander carried in the air were enough to make Mr. Jones gasp for breath.

This story is based on an actual case of an allergy to gerbils, the first one ever reported at a medical meeting.

SKIN TESTS: WHAT'S THE SCORE?

Mr. Jones was lucky in that the cause of his allergy was tracked down rather easily. To detect allergens in other persons from hundreds of possible substances often requires extensive skin tests. These are done after the symptoms, family history, and a thorough physical examination fail to suggest the possible cause. The type of skin test used depends upon whether the skin is scratched lightly or punctured, introducing the allergen *into* and between the layers of the skin.

The first test tried is the *scratch test,* the simplest and safest. Some thirty or forty allergens, sometimes more—animal hairs, various grasses, fish, nuts, wheat—are selected. Each allergen is suspended in a solution. Tiny amounts of allergen are placed in a row on spots on the skin marked off with a blunt instrument. A break is made in the skin. After fifteen minutes, each spot is examined for a reaction. If there is no change, the test is *negative* for that particular allergen. But if a WHEAL, a white bump like a mosquito bite surrounded with a red rim, is formed, it is a *positive* test for that allergen. The test either confirms a suspicion or is helpful in ruling it out.

To make certain that the reaction is due to the allergen and not just to the scratch, a control test is done by placing *only* the solution without allergen on another spot on the skin. This spot should appear the same as in a negative reaction.

The tests may all be negative, or some negative and only some positive, and to different degrees. For example, positive to fish or some shellfish, but not to wheat. Or moderately positive to a special fungus, but strongly positive to horsehair.

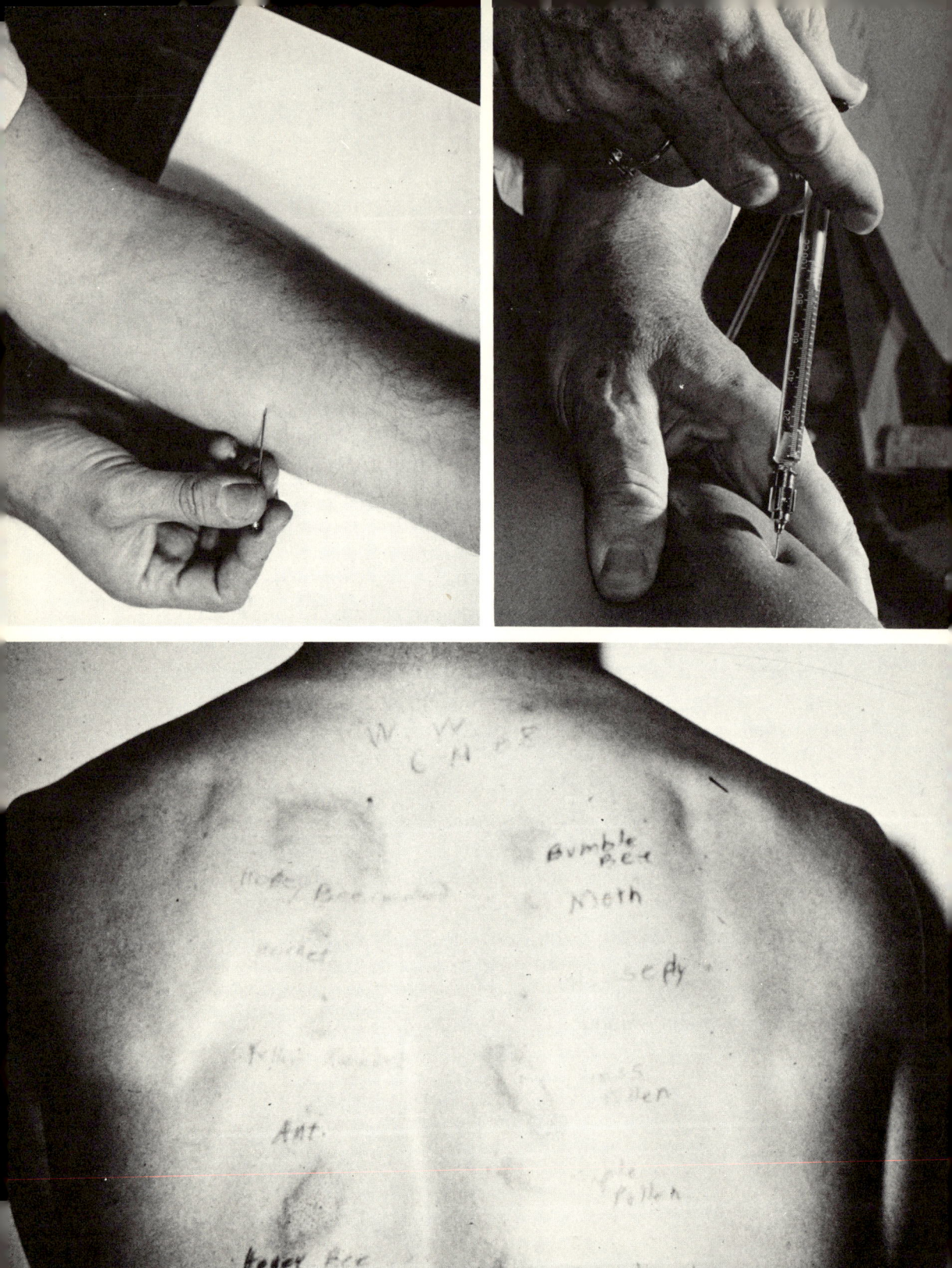

If there is doubt about the results of the scratch test, the allergist may follow up with the *puncture test.* A tiny drop of allergen is injected between the layers of the skin, using a sterile needle. A reaction to an allergen may be negative in the scratch test, but be positive in the puncture test.

TRANSFER TEST

Sometimes the skin test may not be desirable or even possible. The test is then done indirectly through a skin test on another person, a normal (nonsensitive) person. This is the way it is done.

The normal person receives a skin injection of BLOOD SERUM, the watery part of the blood, from the child suspected of having an allergy. The serum contains the antibody against the suspected allergen. Let us say it is wheat. Twenty-four hours later, a tiny amount of wheat allergen, suspended in a solution, is injected into the spot where the presumed antibody-containing serum was injected on the previous day. If a wheal appears in that exact spot, it is a proof that the infant is allergic to wheat. It is like borrowing the antibody from the infant to test it against the allergen in "borrowed" skin. Since the infant is not directly tested, this is called a PASSIVE TRANSFER TEST.

Left: the scratch test
Right: the puncture test
Below: a number of allergens have been applied to this man's back. Several positive reactions appear as wheals.

PATCH TEST

In contact allergy, in which the mere touch of the allergen causes a reaction, the scratch or puncture test is not very useful. In a case like this the suspected allergen is applied to the unbroken skin. Usually, the area is then covered with a moist dressing (a patch) for twenty-four to forty-eight hours. Then the dressing is removed. If a positive reaction appears, as a wheal or a red itching spot, it proves that the substance is the cause of the eruption.

YOUR ALLERGY HAS A NAME

Finding the specific allergen that is causing the trouble is the first big step in treating the allergy. It is really the *diagnosis,* the name that the doctor gives to the trouble. This is how the doctor decides what needs to be done to relieve it.

3

All Clues Lead to Allergic Rhinitis

Barney's mother told the doctor that she couldn't remember Barney being free of "colds," or sniffles, what with his nose being stuffed, or "running a stream." He is a mouth-breather, he snores, his nose sometimes twitches, even in his sleep. During the winter things are worse, she adds. He often coughs, pulls at his ear as if it itches, and now and then he complains of an earache.

Now that Barney is old enough to go to school, there are other problems. He is droopy, and doesn't listen in the classroom. He tires easily, and can't keep up with the other children in outdoor games. His schoolwork suffers because he is absent so often. His appetite is poor and his disposition no better. Little things irritate him. He becomes frustrated when he cannot easily solve a homework problem, just as he is when he doesn't play games well.

Taking down this history of Barney's symptoms, the doctor noted the first telling clue: that the boy kept rubbing his nose up and down—a gesture that allergists have dubbed the "allergic salute."

WHEN DID THE TROUBLE START?

The doctor follows up the list of complaints with the usual

questioning. Did Barney ever have hives? "Come to think of it, yes," his mother remembers—when she first gave him orange juice, and later cream of wheat. At another time, when she dressed him in a woolen sweater and cap, an "angry" rash spread over his face and neck. Did anyone else in the family have complaints like Barney's? Oh yes, she herself had been told that she had allergic bronchitis because of her frequent dry cough, a tightness in the chest, which is worse in the cold, and on windy days. And her sister suffers from migraine headaches, attacks that her doctor says are due to an allergy.

Barney's symptoms and the family history are clues to be followed up by an examination.

WE WILL HAVE A GOOD LOOK AT BARNEY

The doctor looks into the young patient's nose, throat, and ears, at the same time asking more questions, and making a note or two. Is the discharge from his nose always watery or, at times, thick, stringy, or sometimes greenish yellow? Greenish yellow would indicate infection. Allergic children get colds more often than others, and each infection, in turn, makes the allergic symptoms worse. Still, infection as *the* cause must be ruled out.

Looking into the nostrils gives the doctor another clue: the lining is swollen—"boggy," the doctor calls it—and pale to bluish. In an infection the MUCOUS MEMBRANE (the moist lining) is also swollen (CONGESTED, *inflamed*—red). Both infection and allergy would cause sniffles. When an infection clears, the INFLAMMATION and thick yellow discharge disappear. But steady exposure to an allergen would account for the continued watery flow from the swollen membrane.

The swollen membrane obstructs the airway, interfering with normal breathing. This means less oxygen is being delivered to the blood, the nasal lining, and skin. Just so, Barney's face is also pale, and he has dark circles under his eyes. Deficient oxygen could explain his tiredness and irritability.

THEN A SIMPLE TEST

The doctor asks Barney to blow his nose into a piece of wax paper. The doctor spreads a bit of the discharge on a glass slide and puts a drop of dye on it to stain the colorless smear. Under the microscope the doctors sees an excessive number of small white blood cells (now stained with the dye). These cells, called eosinophiles, are the clinching clue to allergy. The same test with the nasal discharge from an infection would show up more of a different kind of white blood cells—the kind that engulf and gobble up bacteria.

Then the doctor listens to Barney's chest. His breathing is shallow, but there is no wheezing. Good! This means that the BRONCHI and branches, the tubes that deliver air to the lungs, are not blocked. But if Barney does not get treatment now, they could become blocked and further interfere with normal breathing. The swollen lining and stuffiness in Barney's nose obstruct the free passage of air to the lungs, making it difficult to breathe through the nose. This is why he breathes through his mouth. Mouth-breathing robs the incoming air of the normal moisture in the nose. It dries the throat and makes him cough.

Barney sometimes complains of an earache. Have his parents or teacher at times suspected that he doesn't hear well? The tube that leads from the throat to the ear is swollen

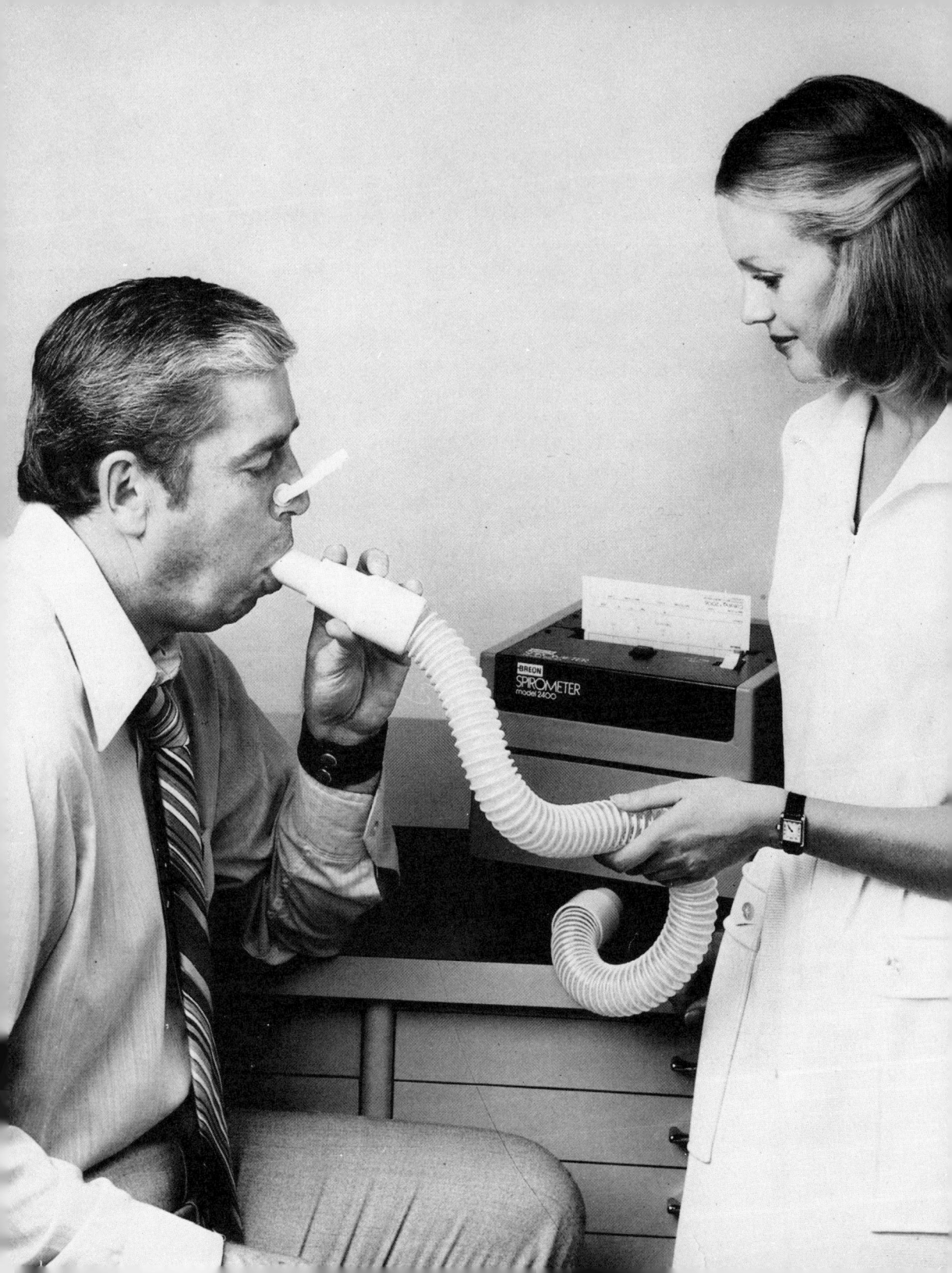

and nearly closed. This could account for his occasional loss of hearing.

The doctor says Barney's trouble is allergic rhinitis. He needs proper care now before his discomfort becomes complicated by nasal growths, called POLYPS, blocked SINUSES (spaces in the facial bones), and enlarged tonsils and adenoids. Such changes only increase the obstruction, making the symptoms worse, and bring other troubles: headaches, repeated infections, and further hearing loss.

WHAT IS BARNEY ALLERGIC TO?

"Does he need skin tests, doctor?" Skin tests are useful and safe, the doctor answers. And if they reveal the exact cause, its removal is the surest way to prevent the troublesome symptoms. But at this time the doctor hesitates to recommend them for Barney, and explains the reasons. Since Barney is not too uncomfortable in the warm seasons of the year, the doctor believes the allergen is probably not pollen. The fact that foods no longer give him hives as in his infancy, means that food is not the cause of his problem.

HOUSE DUST DOES IT

The doctor believes that Barney's rhinitis is caused by one or more airborne allergens. These must be present right in his home, in "house dust." It could be animal dander from pets, insect particles, feathers, and mold spores. Mold allergy,

A spirometer tests the patient's lung function.

for some unknown reason, is especially common in allergic children.

Molds are microscopic, nonflowering plants like mushrooms and other fungi. They live on plants, foods, leather shoes and luggage, dry and decaying leaves, in soil, on textiles, book bindings, and even on old wallpaper. Mold spores are like seeds of other plants. They are easily spread by the wind because of their tiny size and lightness. If they land on warm, humid places, the spores germinate and develop into luxuriant new colonies of mold.

WE CAN MAKE YOU FEEL BETTER

The best way to begin treating mold allergy is to avoid the allergen. But how does one avoid inhaling house dust? Here's the doctor's list of dos and don'ts:

> *Don't* shake bedding, sweep carpets with a broom, or dust furniture with a feather duster.
>
> *Do* use a vacuum cleaner for carpets, hangings, and upholstered furniture. The mold is sucked up in the vacuum bag!
>
> *Don't* sleep on feather or down pillows; avoid wool blankets.
>
> *Do* cover mattresses and all bedding with plastic zippered covers.
>
> *Don't* have wallpaper; use paint instead, or spray the walls with mold-checking material.
>
> *Do* stay away from a dusty garage or attic.
>
> If the cellar is damp, use a dehumidifier to dry it out.

For Barney: NO ANIMAL OR BIRD PETS.

His bedroom should have an airconditioner, window filter, or a gadget called an electrostatic precipitator to screen out the dust.

Protect him against colds and treat an infection promptly.

Avoid crowded, poorly ventilated places.

THERE ARE MEDICINES

For times of special discomfort, the doctor prescribes a medicine—one of a group of drugs called ANTIHISTA-MINES (against histamine). They come in tablets, syrup, as a "nasal mist" (to spray into the nose), drops, or time-release capsules for slow, continued relief.

The medicine shrinks the nasal membrane, eases breathing, and gives relief. It tends to make one sleepy, so it is best used at bedtime for a comfortable night's sleep. But the doctor warns, *don't overdo.* Relief does not last long, and if the medicine is used too often, it may actually cause the swelling to return and be harmful.

If all this should not prove helpful, the doctor may recommend skin tests to identify the exact allergen. Then the next thing is HYPOSENSITIZATION to build up Barney's tolerance to his particular allergen.

4

Hay Fever

IT'S NOT A FEVER

Hay fever sufferers do not run a temperature, so this allergy is not properly called a fever. Nor is freshly mown hay its cause, because by the time the tall grass is harvested, it has passed the sensitizing flowering stage. Some people call it "rose fever," again wrongly. It just happens that roses bloom at about the same time when the inconspicuous flowers of early summer grasses fill the air with pollen. Pollen, which gets its name from the Latin for "fine flour" or "dust," is the yellow mass of powdery sex cells on the STAMEN, the male part of a flower. The doctor's label for hay fever is *seasonal rhinitis,* or POLLINOSIS, which more accurately describes the nature of the allergy and its cause.

Roses and other showy flowers attract insects and birds by their colored petals, scent, and nectar. While gathering their food, bees and birds pick up pollen on their wings and feet, and carry it to the female part of the plant. Hay fever patients may be near these flowers and still enjoy their sweet-smelling odors without distressing symptoms. It is the drab, colorless plants, grasses, weeds, and the hardly noticeable blooms of some trees that release large amounts of light-grained pollen that is carried by the wind. Pollen grains are very small, measuring between twenty-thousandths to forty-thousandths of a millimeter in diameter. (A millimeter is just under four-hundredths [.04] of an inch.) The protein in the pollen grains of wind-pollinated plants is the allergen that causes hay fever. And millions of people have it.

IT'S THAT TIME OF YEAR

Unlike Michael's and Barney's allergy, with symptoms occurring almost any time of the year, hay fever is seasonal. With pretty much the same symptoms, it returns every year during a certain few weeks from spring to fall. In a pollen-sensitive person, the allergic symptoms appear at the same time that the particular offending plant blooms.

THE POLLEN THAT BRINGS THE SNEEZES

Each species of tree produces its own kind of pollen, and its pollination period usually lasts from two to four weeks. In northeastern United States the trees that pollinate late in April to early May are beech, birch, poplar, oak, hickory, ash, maple, cedar, and sycamore. In California and Florida the melaleuca or paper tree blooms in May. In June, it is the early summer grasses: timothy, redtop, orchard grass, Kentucky blue, sorrel and plantain, and certain weeds such as Russian thistle and sagebrush.

   Later in summer and through September ragweed is the plant whose pollen brings the sneezes, runny nose, weeping eyes, and itchy nose, ears, and palate; the nasal mucous membrane swells; breathing is difficult. Ragweed grows luxuriantly in the fall in the east, south, and midwest of United States, but not in the southwest and west of the Rockies. A hay fever sufferer might be comfortable in dry Arizona during the time when the air is full of ragweed pollen in the east.

THE VISIT TO THE ALLERGIST

Uncontrollable spasms of sneezing, especially on arising, itching of the eyes, nose, and throat bring the hay fever victim to the allergist. These distressful symptoms are worse while playing outside, riding in an open car, or when camping out. They are worse on windy days, and not as bad during wet weather. This is all familiar to the allergist. As with other allergies, hayfever is believed to be a family susceptibility. But the single most important clue to correctly identifying the cause is the seasonal history.

Going on from there, the allergist has some diagnostic aids. He or she consults a chart that shows the kinds of vegetation in the patient's geographical locality. The allergy area map shows where and when each kind of allergic plant blooms. A pollen count chart tells the pollen density in different locations, even at different altitudes at certain times of the year. The number of pollen grains of each species can be counted under the microscope.

First the pollen count. Pollen is collected by exposing a glass slide for a specific period at different locations. Then the density of grains of each variety is estimated under the microscope. The pollen count of each of the grains is reported as a given number present per cubic yard of air.

Then the type of pollen. The pollen grain of each species can be recognized, again under the microscope.

With these aids and by questioning the patient, the allergist tries to track down the allergen. Does the onset of symptoms coincide with and last for the certain weeks shown on the chart in the patient's locality?

HOW DOES IT WORK?

We need to begin with where the allergen provokes the reaction in an allergic person. The body produces the antibody, a protein that belongs to a class of molecules called IMMUNOGLOBULINS. The particular one in this class, involved in allergy, is Immunoglobulin E, usually written as *IgE*. When IgE combines with the allergen, such as ragweed pollen, it acts on the surface of special cells, known as mast cells, and disrupts the cell membrane, releasing histamine. Histamine acts on the shock organs; in this case on the mucous lining of the nose, bringing on sneezing and itching. It also causes the capillaries (the tiny thin-walled blood vessels) to widen and leak fluid into the tissues, causing them to swell. The accumulation of this fluid is known as edema.

    The purpose of hyposensitization is gradually to block this reaction by the repeated injection of allergen. This allows the patient to build up tolerance to it. Does this block the allergic antibody, or does it produce some other substance that competes with it? Just how this happens is not really known, but it does work. For ragweed it is now possible to measure the amount of the antigen necessary to bind the IgE antibody. What's more, since IgE can be removed from the blood serum, and its chemistry understood, it is possible that it can be altered, so that when injected it will block the allergic reaction.

THE TIME MAY COME

A research scientist has discovered that a small portion of

the IgE molecule (a very tiny unit) is what blocks the allergic reaction. This part of it has been synthesized in the laboratory. It is made up of only five amino acids, the building blocks of proteins. Complete proteins are much more complicated. This prepared chemical is like a split-off IgE. When injected it seems to reduce the allergic reaction. Since it is digested in the stomach, it cannot be taken as a tablet, but must be injected. Much more work has to be done.

Another development has been reported from Germany. Seventy children, aged three to thirteen years, who were allergic to pollen were given one drop of a very weak dilution of the allergen extract prepared with glycerine. Peppermint was added to make it tastier. It had to be taken on an empty stomach. The treatment was given three times a week during the winter to desensitize the children before the hay fever season. It seems to have worked for those children.

All this is something for the future. In the meantime, without hyposensitization, and if complete avoidance is not possible, doctors prescribe the same medicines for hay fever as for perennial allergic rhinitis. The warnings against overuse are the same.

5

Asthma

WHEN IT'S HARD TO BREATHE

Lori, who is twelve, has had ASTHMA since she was three years old. If you asked her what her misery is, she would be quick to say: "It's so hard to breathe." No wonder *asthma* is the Greek word for "panting"! During those years she was treated with medicines that relieved her wheezing, labored breathing, and tight feeling in the chest. But there were times when that was not enough. Things were often so bad that she not only had to stay out of school but needed to be in a hospital for vigorous and frequent emergency treatment.

In asthma the shock organ is the lung. Here is what happens to obstruct the air passages. Normally, air freely enters the lungs from the bronchi through many of their branches that finally end in tiny tubes, the BRONCHIOLES. The bronchioles are ringed with muscle tissue. In asthma the muscle rings contract, narrowing the opening. It is then difficult for air to pass in and out of the lungs. The wheezing is due to the forced exit of air on breathing out. Air becomes trapped in the lungs, causing them to overinflate. In fact, this enlargement of the lungs eventually changes the shape of the chest, and even makes the heart seem smaller than normal.

The trapped air picks up the carbon dioxide gas wastes that the body gives off, which cannot readily leave the narrowed bronchioles, just as oxygen in the entering fresh air cannot fully ventilate the lungs. As a result, the blood carries less than the normal amount of oxygen and more than the normal amount of carbon dioxide. The very effort to ventilate the lungs makes matters worse, as it takes more energy to breathe. In a severe attack, eating, talking, or laughing may be too much of an effort. The skin begins to turn blue. Lying down is worse than sitting up.

Other changes take place. The bronchiolar walls swell and the tubes fill with an extra amount of MUCUS, formed by the bronchial glands. This tends to plug up the tubes. Coughing is the body's way of ridding the tubes of the mucus. As in other allergies, eosinophiles, those special white blood cells, invade the bronchiolar wall.

THE ASTHMATIC PERSONALITY

If the physical handicap isn't bad enough, the asthmatic child has other problems that interfere with developing a normal healthy and happy nature. The child loses confidence, shows little initiative, shrinks from taking part in activities with schoolmates, is unhappy, feels lost, and is overly dependent on adults. Feeling left out, the child may demand extra attention from parents, often becomes aggressive and bullies other children. All because of a distressing disease!

Children with chronic (long-lasting) asthma, who needed the special help provided in a hospital and research center in Denver, Colorado, were encouraged to speak their troubled minds in sessions with sympathetic adults on the staff.

What did they really feel? Both boys and girls expressed anger, envy, sadness, fear of being scolded, or guilt for upsetting their parents. Some resented their healthy brothers and sisters, others were frightened of harsh-sounding teachers. Some said they felt like "pin cushions" from all the injections, or as "guinea pigs" given medicine that "didn't do much good anyway." One felt guilty because his sister had to give up a dog because of his allergy. Clearly, these asthmatic children need a great deal of patient understanding because their troubles are very real, and constant.

A COMBINATION OF CAUSES

When and how did it all start? Allergists agree that three out of four children of allergic parents may begin sneezing, and maybe wheezing, any time before they are ten years old, most by the time they reach school age. Of all the allergies, asthma is the most serious in children. It occurs about five to seven times as often in children than in adults. And about a third of the children who get asthma have a history of ECZEMA in the first year or two, as in Lori's case. As an infant she was afflicted with the scaly, crusty, sometimes oozing skin, and was always itchy.

Usually the eczema clears, and only somewhat later does the asthma show up. It is now thought that the first attack may occur after a virus infection of the respiratory system (breathing system) during the fall and winter influenza season. Blood tests have led doctors to suspect a link between such an infection and an allergic attack. Tests showed that more histamine and IgE were in the blood in allergic children after an infection than before.

More than likely it is more than one kind of allergen that causes asthma: one or more foods, inhalants, pollen, and animal dander. Even a blast of cold air, or a chemical or mechanical irritant in the air could trigger an attack. Coal dust, chalk dust, flying ash, smoke, or sulfur chemicals in polluted air may also cause a sudden spasm of the bronchioles in an asthmatic child.

MORE THAN ONE WAY OF RELIEF

Experience sometimes reveals *the* offending allergen. In that lucky case, avoidance of it can help prevent the onset of symptoms. If it cannot be avoided, the remedy is gradual hyposensitization, as in hay fever. Relief may also be achieved by medicines that get at the distressing symptoms. From antihistamines to aerosols the drugs work to dilate (open up) the narrowed bronchioles. They make breathing easier by relaxing muscle spasms of the bronchioles. These drugs are given by mouth, by spray, by injection, or by rectal suppository for relief during sleep. For young or frightened children, a sedative or calming drug may be necessary. In a severe attack epinephrine, also called adrenalin, is injected for more prompt relaxation of the muscle in the bronchioles. It may even be necessary to put the child into an oxygen tent, or be helped to breathe by a machine that supplies oxygen by pressure through a tube.

To help unplug the tubes of mucus, an expectorant drug that reduces the thickness of mucus is given. Still another

The lung is the shock organ in asthma. A hand nebulizer is used during an asthma attack.

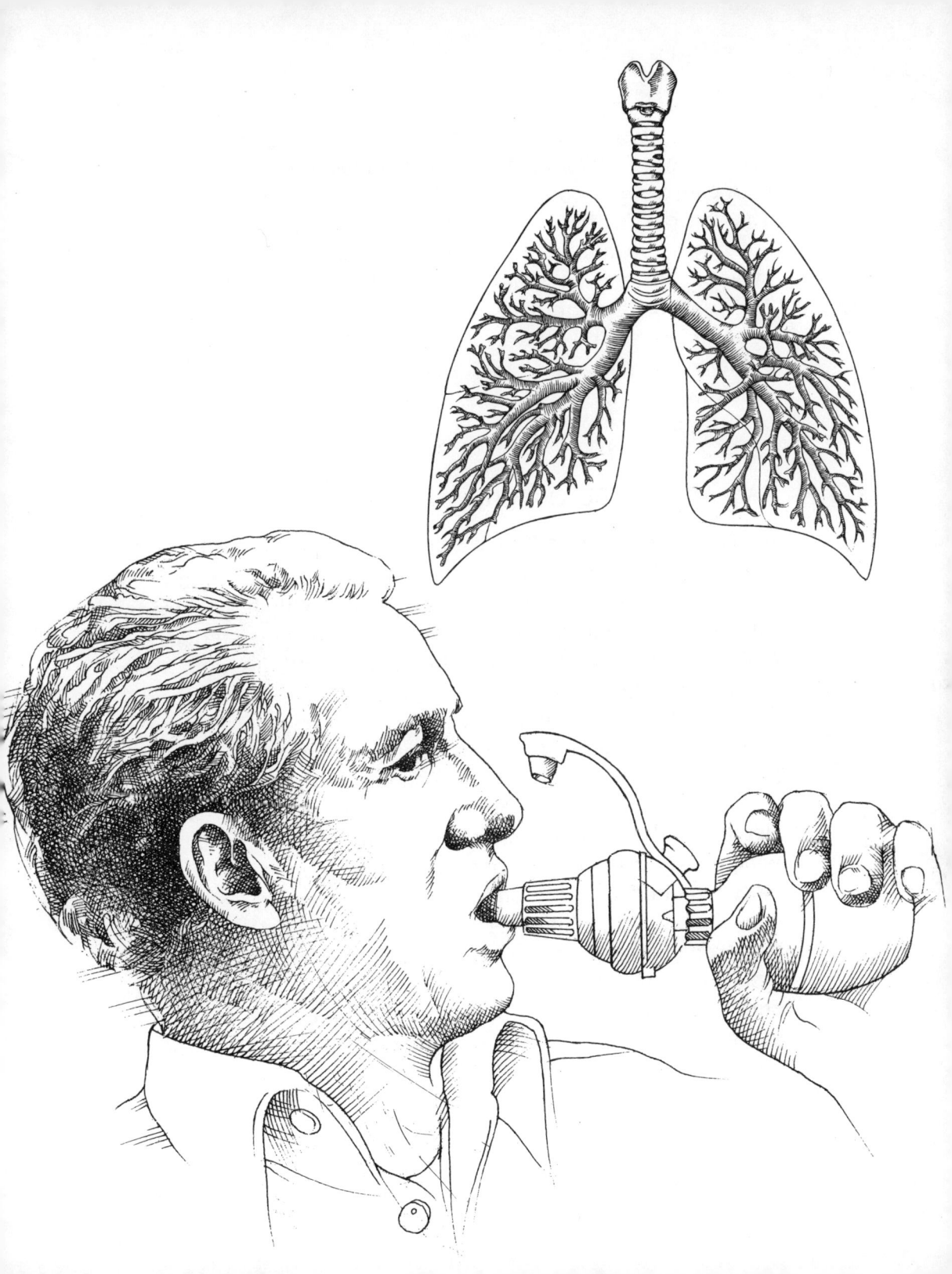

group of drugs called corticosteroids are used in chronic cases. These substances are hormones normally produced by a gland in the body. They are also made in the laboratory. The trouble is that they tend to retard growth, as well as cut down the natural production by the body. So they are avoided as long as other medicines relieve the symptoms, and prevent damage to the lungs. In recent years they have been replaced by newer drugs. One of these, cromolyn, actually prevents an attack. The way it acts is to check the breakdown of the mast cells, thereby preventing the release of histamine.

CAN ASTHMA BE OUTGROWN?

Allergies are not cured, as we know. Still, about half the children who have been treated stop wheezing and seem to have "outgrown" their troublesome symptoms in their late teens. The younger the child and the sooner treatment is started, the better are the chances of improvement and freedom from symptoms. They may then look forward to a normal happy life. However, long and drawn-out care is required, but it should not be neglected. The alternative is stunted growth, permanent damage to the lungs, and the life of an invalid.

    Lori is lucky because she received proper treatment. Her breathing is improving. The amount of air she takes in each breath is rising. She gets enough oxygen to do the exercises required of other children—all because her medicines have helped to reduce the severity and frequency of asthmatic attacks. Her doctor says that like so many other asthmatic patients she should continue to improve. About 50 percent tend to become free of symptoms before they are twenty years old, and about one-third more are improved later in life.

6

When Food Is the Allergen

Most people can eat almost any food. But for some people one or more foods, even in the tiniest amounts, may cause frightening symptoms. A food allergy can show up at any age, and often occurs in babies.

THE TROUBLED BABY

In some infants the allergy affects the skin in the form of eczema and lasts for a year or more. It seems that breast-fed babies are generally immune, while those fed on a formula are more likely to get it. Eczema is extremely rare in underdeveloped countries, in Africa and Asia, and more prevalent in industrialized countries such as the United States. Perhaps this is because, with few exceptions, infants are breast-fed in underdeveloped countries. And because the range of foods in the diet of the adults of underdeveloped countries is more limited and stable.

    Eczema usually starts two or three months after birth, and the skin eruption has an easily recognizable pattern. First it shows up on the face, neck, ears, and scalp; then inside the forearm and at the elbow bends. Later it spreads to the front of the trunk and legs. During the second year it moves to the back of the trunk and knees.

The eczematous skin is red, covered with "weeping" (oozing) blisters, crusts, and scales. The upper layers of the skin thicken. The terrible itching leads to scratching, which makes the condition worse and often leads to infection. If cow's milk is thought to be the cause, goat's milk or special formulas, such as soybean preparations, are substituted. Sometimes boiling the milk will help, by changing the protein in such a way that it is no longer allergenic.

Treating the skin directly is another problem. Irritating soaps and overdressing, which would cause excessive sweating, should be avoided. To prevent scratching, the nails are cut short and the skin is covered with bandages over a layer of ointments, sometimes containing cortisone.

Allergic infants may not get eczema. The target organ could be the stomach or intestine. The baby may be colicky, have cramps and diarrhea, and regurgitate (spit up) its food. Since an infant's diet consists of relatively few foods, it is easier to find the one causing the trouble. Usually one new food is introduced at a time. If the baby reacts badly to it, it should be eliminated from its diet.

SYMPTOMS GALORE

The symptoms of food allergy in adults may involve many parts of the body. Sneezing, wheezing, stuffiness; swelling around the eyes, lips, face, and tongue; cramps, nausea, vomiting, diarrhea; migraine headaches; and URTICARIA (hives) over the entire body, which takes the form of raised patches, either red or pale, and terrible itching.

Tracking down a food allergen in an adult is much more difficult than in an infant. Adults eat a wider variety of foods. Sometimes a food taken in very small quantities will cause no reaction, but will produce hives when eaten in larger amounts. Even the time of year may make a difference. If during the berry or peach season a person eats these in quantity, the allergy will show up, where it wouldn't cause any trouble from a single strawberry added to a dessert at Christmas. The reaction sometimes is immediate, almost before the food is even swallowed. At other times, the reaction is delayed for a couple of days. How would you remember what you ate? Also, the offending allergen may not be the whole food, but rather the product of digestion, or otherwise changed.

For these reasons, a food allergy is one of the hardest to track down. Skin tests are rarely helpful, not only because of the large number of possible allergens, but also because extracts are difficult to prepare and are unstable. So we have to look to other means.

ELIMINATION AND CHALLENGE

To begin with, the allergist may suggest keeping a food diary: list all the foods eaten each day for a week, then write down on what day a reaction occurred. Let's say that food X is the one suspected. Suppose it is chocolate that the patient thinks triggered the reaction. Then the allergist would say, "Stay away from chocolate for two weeks." Of course, that means not only candy, but chocolate soda, cocoa, and chocolate cookies.

If during this period of eliminating chocolate there were no symptoms, the doctor may then suggest trying a small amount of it. This is called the "challenging" procedure. If the symptoms reappear on challenge, then this is considered a positive test: allergic to chocolate! From then on the person should continue to eliminate it from the diet. But it may not always be that easy.

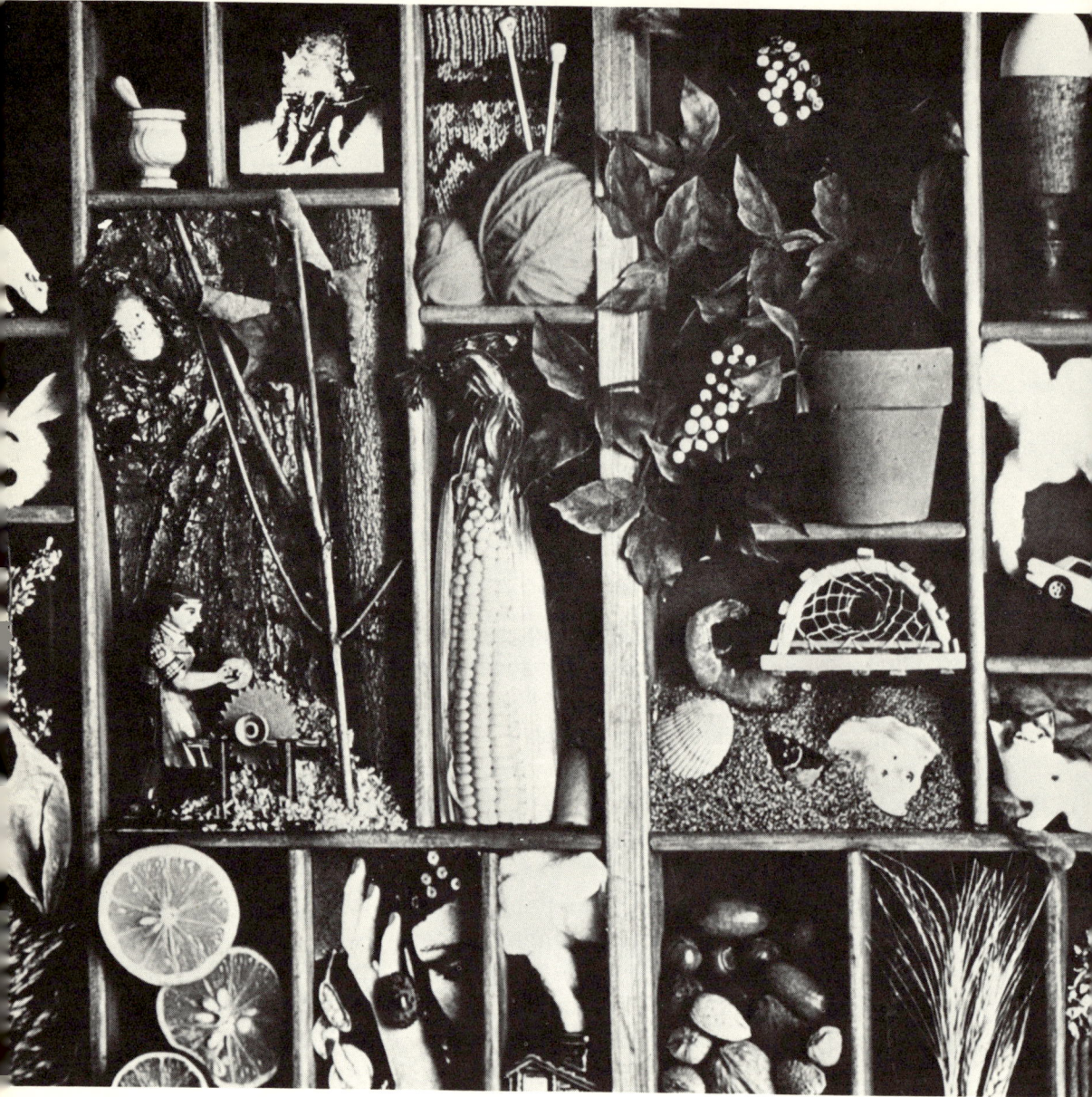

Another method has been tried with a number of patients known to have food and other allergies. (It often happens that persons allergic to one or more foods are also pollen sensitive, for example.) They were given what is called a *synthetic, nonallergenic diet,* the kind given to patients who have had surgery, have an opening from the stomach to the outside, or have suffered severe burns. The diet contains amino acids, instead of whole proteins, sugar, minerals, and vitamins. The patients were not to eat or drink anything else, except water. If the cause of their allergy was a food, they had complete relief within a week. If the cause was a pollen or mold, this diet made no difference; their symptoms remained. For those with a food allergy, suspected foods were added, one at a time, along with the synthetic diet until the offending one was revealed by an allergic reaction.

To make things even more complicated, it sometimes happens that people have allergic reactions to foods they haven't even *eaten,* just *smelled.* One patient in this group was a restaurant waitress. She took a two-week leave, staying at home and living on the synthetic diet. When she returned to work, still sticking to her diet, she became violently ill. The doctor was then sure that it was not what she ate, but the food vapors she inhaled in the restaurant that made her sick.

HIVES FROM OTHER CAUSES

Urticaria may be caused other than by allergens. People under severe emotional stress may break out in a rash. Some

*All sorts of substances cause
allergic reactions in some people.*

children may develop a rash suddenly and seemingly without cause. It may appear to be a trick, but when they are upset by their parents they get a rash. It is really their disappointment or anger that shows up by blotches on the skin.

There are other people whose skin is so sensitive that just stroking it with a blunt object will make the lines stand out as a series of wheals with reddened borders. Although nothing is eaten or inhaled, it is still an allergic reaction, a *physical* allergy. It is called DERMATOGRAPHISM, from the Greek meaning to "write on the skin." You may not believe it, but it is possible to write such a person's name on his or her back, just by spelling it out with your finger.

DRUG SENSITIVITY

It need not be a food, but a drug. Prescription drugs carry a warning that its use should be discontinued if the person shows a sensitivity to it. A drug that most people tolerate well may cause one person in many thousands to get hives or some other reaction.

One drug given, not as a medication to treat a disease but to make a diagnosis, makes an internal organ stand out on X-ray film. A small number of people develop a reaction a day or two after swallowing it. One very dangerous reaction is swollen mouth, tongue, and throat. If not immediately treated with a corticosteroid, it could cause suffocation.

7

Don't Let a Bee Sting Again

Stings by bees, wasps, hornets, and yellow jackets are not new, rare, or to be ignored. The HIEROGLYPHICS (picture writing) on Egyptian tablets tell that King Menes, the legendary first king of Egypt, died from the sting of a hornet. That was in 2641 B.C. In the United States, a recent five-year record showed that more people died from stinging insects than from snake bites. This is reason enough to beware of what could be a life threatening emergency.

NOT IN THE FAMILY

Unlike other allergies, a severe reaction to an insect sting may occur to someone who has no allergies, and who has no family history of allergy. The first time the person is stung, there may be only a local reaction. The spot of the sting reddens, swells slightly, and hurts due to an acid secreted. The real damage is that this first sting injects venom that sensitizes the person to a second sting some time later. The venom comes from a pair of the insect's glands and is contained in a venom or poison sac. It is the venom that releases histamine, which produces the redness, swelling, and itching. In the case of a bee, the stinger will remain in the flesh of the person stung. It is most important to remove the stinger immediately with tweezers, and to flick off the venom sac taking care not to mash it. An ice bag or a couple of ice cubes placed on the spot helps to reduce the local reaction. If the sting is on the arm or leg, the limb should be raised and rested. Better yet, a tourniquet placed *above* the site of the sting (between the wound and the heart) will lessen the spread of the venom.

DANGER: THE SECOND STING!

One doctor warned a mother when her child had a severe reaction to an insect sting: "The next sting might be her last." (Only eight-tenths of one percent [0.8%] of the population are sensitive to such stings, but each year about forty deaths occur among them, according to the United States Bureau of Vital Statistics.) In a sensitized person the reaction is *systemic*, because the symptoms involve nearly all systems of the body. Here is the frightening list: itching and swelling around the eyes and face, dry hacking cough, tightness of the throat and chest, hives all over, labored breathing, hoarseness and difficult speech, chills and fever, fast heart beat, low blood pressure—total shock. It all comes on so quickly that only emergency treatment at a hospital can save the person. The reaction is called ANAPHYLACTIC SHOCK, from the Greek words meaning "without protection."

TO THE EMERGENCY ROOM

Cindy's home was surrounded by trees, bushes, and flower-

This bumblebee uses its long tongue to get nectar from flowers.

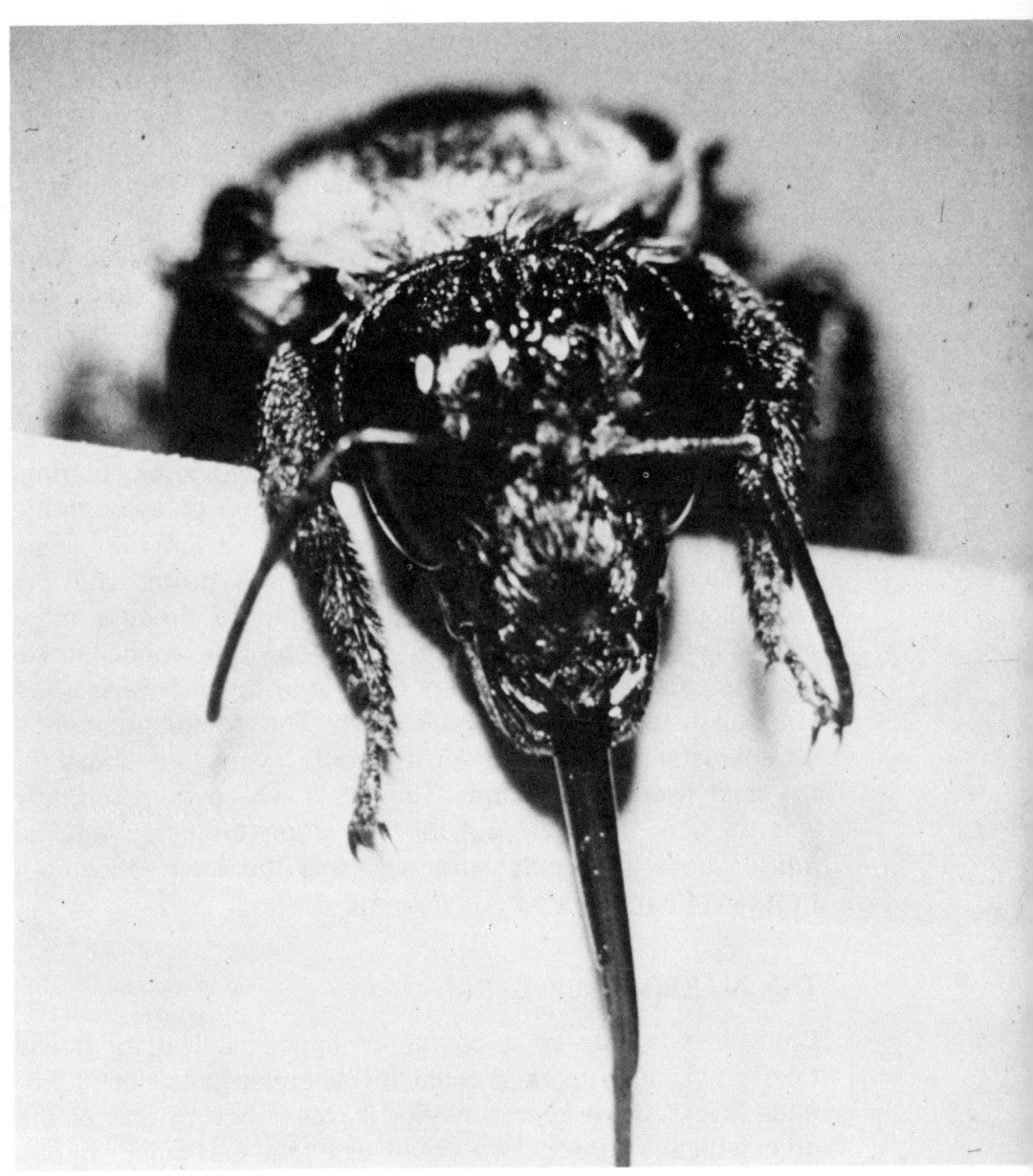

beds. Stinging insects flitted from flower to flower. Hornet nests hung under the eaves of the house and behind the window shutters. Yellow jackets built their nests in spaces between the brick walls. Cindy was five years old when one day she ran into the house screaming that she had been stung by a bee again. It was only two weeks after her first sting.

Cindy's doctor could not be reached, and her eyes were already beginning to swell. There was no time to lose. Her mother called the police station. When the officer arrived he recognized the trouble at once when he saw the bloated face and the pained effort to breathe. He called the hospital to alert them that he was bringing a patient with a severe reaction to an insect sting. And off they went with sirens blaring.

Immediately Cindy received an injection of epinephrine and the doctors watched her breathing and felt her pulse. Within ten minutes, another injection was given, and the bronchiolar spasm relaxed. Cindy began to breathe more easily. This was followed by an injection of an antihistamine into the muscle, and gradually Cindy's symptoms waned and she began to look like herself again. The doctor prescribed an antihistamine to be taken by mouth every four hours for the next twenty-four hours. The crisis was over and Cindy was as good as ever. But, *she must be protected against future stings.* The only sure way was the long, drawn-out process of building up her immunity.

THE ALLERGIST EXPLAINS

Cindy has to receive a course of hyposensitization. It will take a long time to raise what the allergist calls her "tolerance level." If we knew whether it was a bee or one of the other stinging insects, we could use that particular venom.

But it's hard to be sure which one produced the sting. Instead, what is used is an extract of the whole body of the four stinging insects. The smallest possible dose of extract—one-hundred-millionth (1/100,000,000) as much as in a sting—is injected into the skin—just enough to cause a red spot, no more than an inch across. Cindy has to remain at least fifteen minutes in the office, to make certain that there is no other reaction.

The injection has to be repeated every week for about two months, as judged by the reaction, then every two weeks, finally every month. Each time the dose is increased ever so slightly, making sure that the dose is tolerated. How long will this take? How many visits to the doctor? The doctors cannot be sure, but at least three years. Sometimes the person finds out after another sting. If the reaction is only local, it should be treated with an ice bag and antihistamine for twenty-four hours. If a systemic reaction sets in, then it means rushing to the hospital again.

THE TAG AND KIT THAT MAY SAVE YOUR LIFE

Anyone who has had one severe systemic reaction should always wear a wrist or neck tag. It reads: "I am allergic to insect stings." All drugstores have these official tags. Also, the child's health record in school should have a note of the sensitivity, with instructions about whom to call. In case of emergency, if the parent or the doctor cannot be reached, the child should be taken to the nearest hospital.

But suppose you are on a camping trip or somewhere miles away from a hospital or physician? The insect sting kit is the answer. Scout leaders, school nurses, lifeguards, and

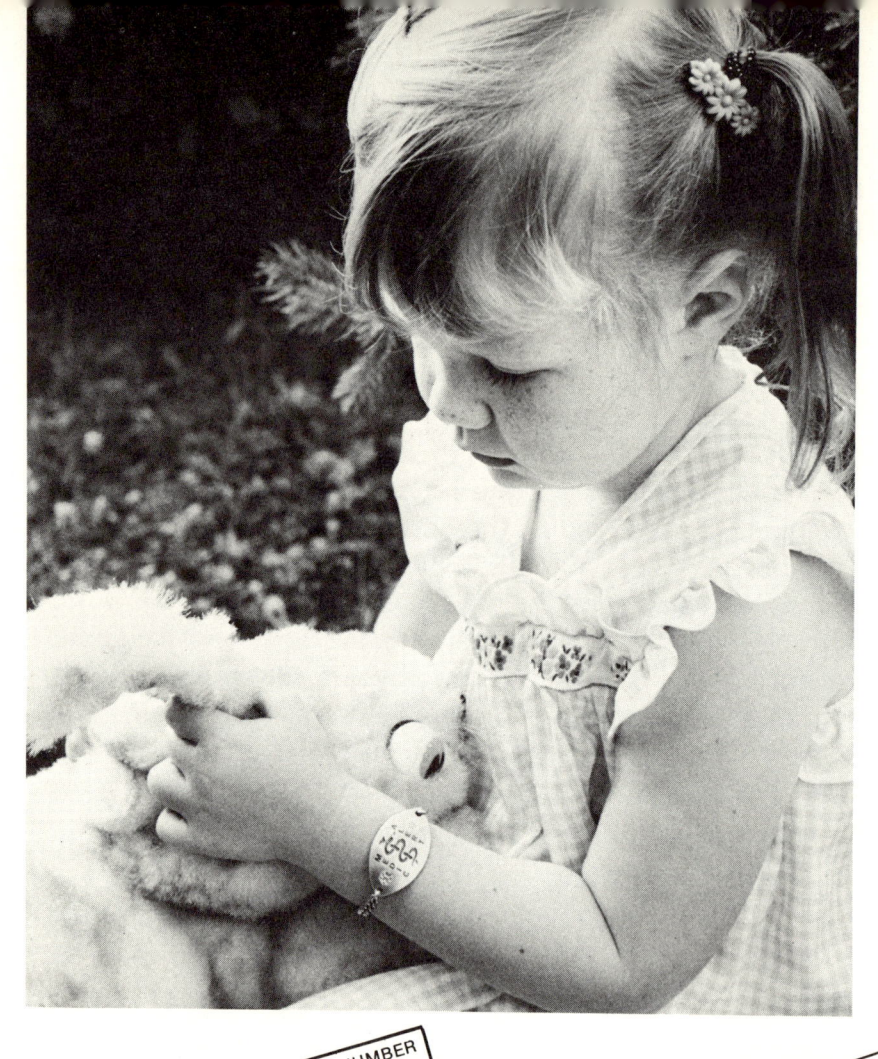

MEDIC ALERT MEMBER INFORMATION
MEMBER NUMBER 00000000

Carter, Laura Ann
483 Giradeau Drive   (615) 395-7849
La Follette TN
                IN AN EMERGENCY CALL
                        (615) 395-7849
Walter Carter   (615)
William Janeway, M.D.
            MY MEDICAL PROBLEM IS

ALLERGIC TO HORSE SERUM

IN AN EMERGENCY CALL COLLECT (209) 6

MEDIC ALERT MEMBER INFORMATION
MEMBER NUMBER 6548369

SMITH, MARY JANE
7605 PARK AVE   (212) 634-1987
NEW YORK, NY 11554   (212) 687-1492
              IN AN EMERGENCY CALL
                       (212) 634-1987
DR THOMAS JOHNSON
GERALD SMITH
          MY MEDICAL PROBLEM IS

DIABETES
HEART CONDITION
WEARING CONTACT LENSES
)TAKES NPH U100 INSULIN, DIGOXIN
DATE ISSUED 6/10/76

IN AN EMERGENCY CALL COLLECT (209) 634-49

forest rangers should have one as a regular item in first aid supplies. The insect-sensitive person should have one at home. It will provide emergency treatment on the spot.

What's in the kit? Here is a list: tweezers, a tourniquet, several sterile gauze pads for swabbing, antihistamine tablets, epinephrine inhaler for difficult breathing, a syringe loaded with epinephrine ready to use for injection, instructions that are simple enough for any level-headed person to follow, and a couple of tranquilizer capsules to soothe a frightened child. Doctors say the insect kit buys time in a life-or-death emergency, until a doctor is at hand.

SOMETHING NEW—IN THE FUTURE

Hyposensitization with the whole body extract is a long and tedious process, and the amount and kind difficult to establish. It would be nice if the venom itself of each of the separate stinging insects was available. An allergist, in experiments with wasp venom obtained from the wasp's venom sac, injected the venom in steadily increasing doses over a period of five hours *in one day.* Within a year, the patient returned for a booster dose. In several hundred patients she has tested the immunity with a challenge sting by an insect *itself,* and found that 85 percent of her patients had excellent resistance for up to three and a half years. The rest had mild reactions to the sting. But more study is needed, the doctor says. Hyposensitization with venom instead of body extract is still in the future.

Above: wearing a Medic Alert tag may save this young girl's life in an emergency.
Below: Medic Alert also issues identification cards to be carried at all times.

8

Is It Something You Touched?

Suppose some part of the skin became red, irritated, and itchy. The doctor may call it CONTACT DERMATITIS, an inflammation of the skin (from the Greek word *dermat,* meaning "skin"). It is not a true allergy. Unlike pollen or animal dander the offending substance is not an allergen; it does not trigger the release of histamine in the body. The reaction is not immediate but is delayed for hours and sometimes for a day or more. This is why it is called delayed hypersensitivity. Also you do not inherit the susceptibility to contact dermatitis from your family. The local reaction is caused by touching certain plants, animal products, or by coming in contact with any one of many chemicals around us. The reaction is usually restricted to the point of contact with the skin.

POISON IVY

Poison ivy is a low-growing weed, although a climbing type grows on fences, rocks, or trees. It has a three-branched waxy leaf and white berries. Some people think that just being *near* poison ivy will give them the inflammation. Not true.

A poison ivy plant

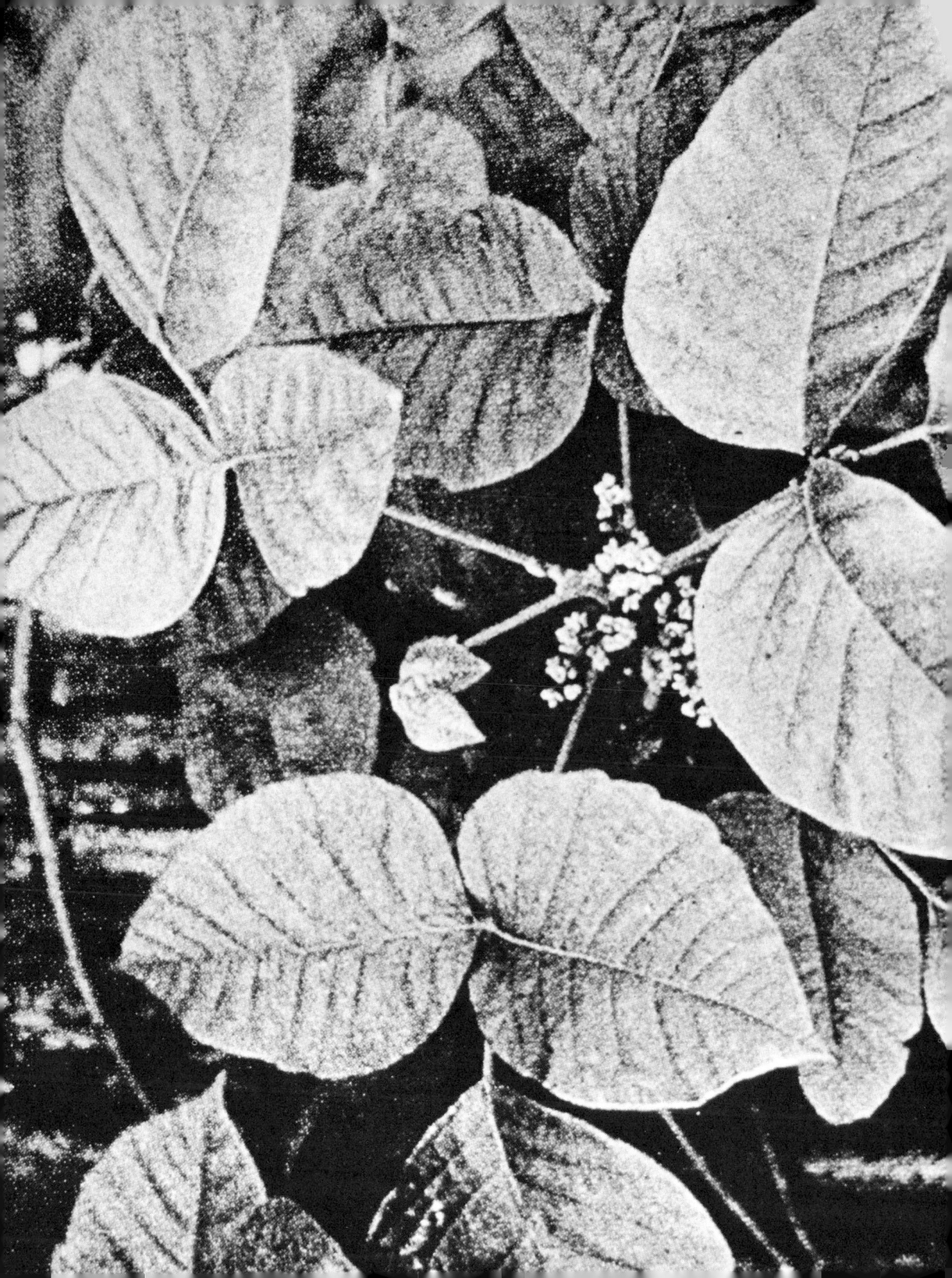

It must actually be touched. Without knowing it, people often brush against the leaves or twigs. The red blebs appear in a line on the skin, as if the poison were streaked. This arrangement, in fact, identifies the eruption as being most likely poison ivy. You could also get it if you petted a dog after it rolled around in a patch of poison ivy. The rash and severe itching may not appear for a day or more after contact. A wise precaution is to scrub the skin with a detergent soap after an outing in the woods, just in case you have come in contact with the plant.

WHAT TO DO

To relieve the itching apply a soothing antihistaminic lotion or calomine lotion with phenol, both of which are sold in the drugstore. AVOID SCRATCHING; it may cause infection when the blisters are broken. If there is swelling and oozing, apply a compress soaked in Burow's solution. If the irritation is widespread because you have sat or lain in a poison ivy patch, you may need a doctor to prescribe an antihistaminic to take by mouth, or an ointment containing HYDROCORTISONE (of the corticosteroid family) applied to the affected area.

KNOW THE PLANT

The best way to avoid poison ivy is to learn how to recognize the plant. Stay out of areas where you see it growing. If it should be growing in your backyard, around the ball park, or anywhere people can't easily avoid it, it should be dug up. Like all weeds, it is persistent and will grow again unless the area is thoroughly cleared. It can also be removed with a weed killer. Removal by burning is not advised because the irritant may be carried in the smoke and affect sensitive persons. If you never again come in contact with it, you will not get another case of poison ivy in your life. Remember it is not a true allergy.

A CHEMIST ON THE TRACK OF A REMEDY

A chemist at the University of Mississippi may have stumbled on something to prevent the poison ivy rash. Its poisonous chemical is an irritant called *urushiol*. The chemist thought that if somehow it could be dissolved and washed away, the battle would be won. So he searched around in the soil where the plant grew, and found bacteria that produce an enzyme that breaks down the oil, the way food is broken down by enzymes in the body. He grew the bacteria in a glass dish in the laboratory, and then extracted the enzyme they produced.

To test how it would work, the chemist brushed the plant across his skin to give himself a case of poison ivy. Then he put some of the bacterial product on one spot, but not on another patch of the skin. The treated area stayed free of the rash. The untreated (control) area blossomed with the expected itching rash. More trials are needed to see if it really works all the time. So don't count on it yet.

LOADS OF CHEMICALS IN OUR LIFE

In our modern world we are surrounded with countless substances that contain chemical irritants with which we come in daily contact. Some can produce a contact dermatitis. We touch them, put them on our faces, work with them, use them for cleaning, patching, repairing, or wear them as part of clothing. Such irritants may be contained in hair coloring,

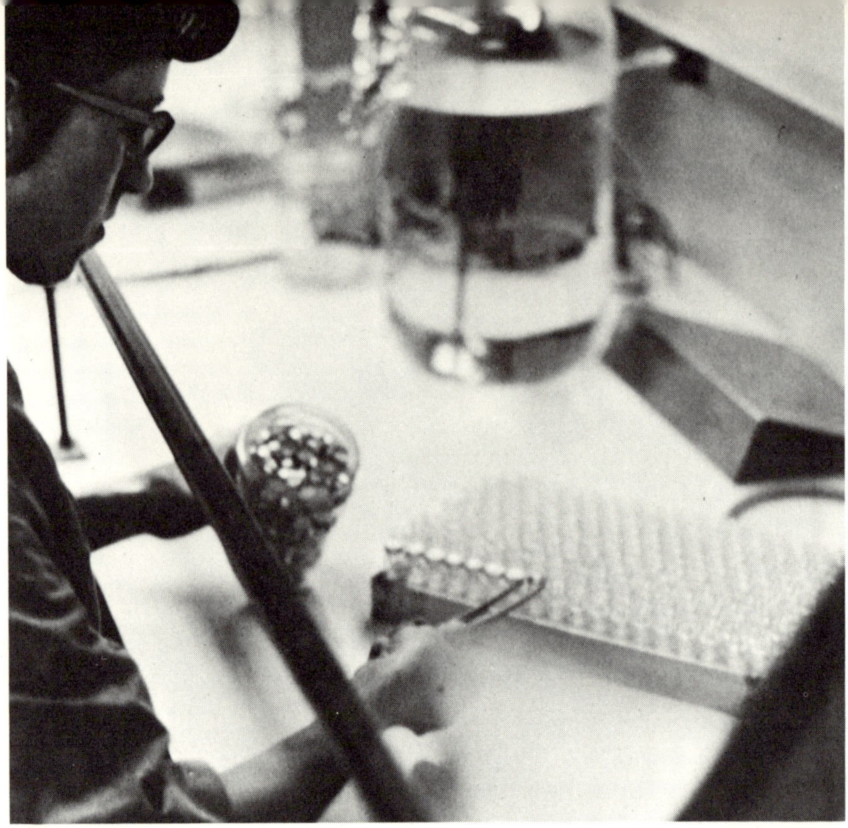

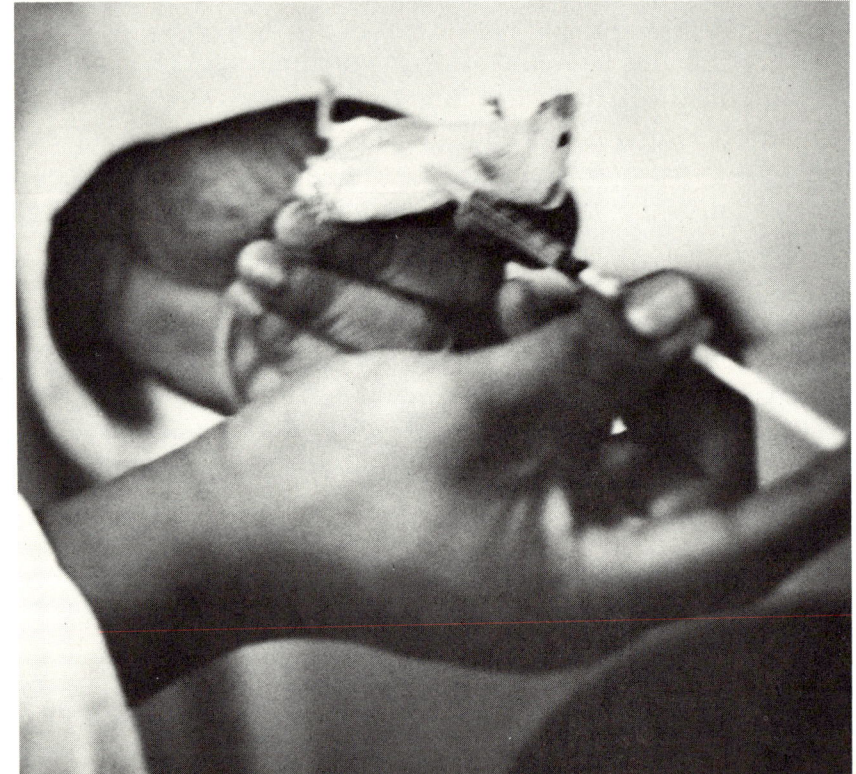

shampoos, deodorants, antiperspirants, face powder, lipstick, eye shadow, nail polish and nail polish remover, bubble bath salts, perfumes, and drugs contained in cosmetic ointments and creams. Then there are sprays or dusts on fruits or vegetables treated with pesticides, inks, carbon paper, rubber cement, waxed cartons, dyes, paints, lacquers, varnishes, and turpentine. Irritants exist in some textiles—acetate, nylon (usually when the garment is new)—plastics, antibiotics, certain metals—in costume jewelry—chrome, and mercury. Here is an example of mercury as an irritant in one case. A woman who was sensitive to antiseptics that contained mercury accidentally broke a thermometer one day and touched a drop of the spilled mercury. Within hours she broke out in a rash.

After repeated contact, some people may become sensitized to one or more of these chemicals, while most people may never get a reaction to the same chemical. To find out which one produced a rash is often a frustrating detective job. It is not as easy as in the case of the woman who was known to be sensitive to mercury.

When the rash appears, one has to think back to check what new or different substance one came in contact with. When the rash is limited to one spot it helps to track it down. Was it a new lipstick, or deodorant? If the mouth or underarms are the areas affected, the job of detection is made easier. The suspected item can then be checked by the patch test. Once the offending substance is identified, the remedy is avoidance.

Preparing vaccines for allergies is careful and important work. Vaccines are tested on animals before they are used on people.

NOT ALL DRUG REACTIONS ARE ALLERGIC

Penicillin is one of the few and best-known drugs to cause a true allergic reaction in some people. As with other chemicals, we have today many thousands of new drugs that did not exist fifty years ago. They are prescribed to many millions of people. The same drug given to an untold number of patients will produce no ill effects. But one in a great number of persons may react badly to it, with nausea, cramps, ringing in the ears, or some other discomfort. That person is said to have a sensitivity or IDIOSYNCRASY to the particular drug. In that case the patient is taken off the offending drug, and another for the same disease substituted. An idiosyncrasy is not a true allergic reaction, but a rare individual occurrence. Still it must not be ignored.

Contact dermatitis is a problem of modern life, because we are today immersed in a sea of chemicals. And they are foreign to the body, which is why some people react to them. When the cause of allergy—true allergy—was discovered in 1905 by two young Austrian doctors, it was through the body's reaction to foreign blood serum. In fact, the title of their book, translated from the German, was *Serum Sickness.* In sufficient amounts serum produced anaphylactic shock in animals. It is an allergen in humans too, just as is any foreign substance introduced into the blood.

In the course of thousands of years, allergies such as asthma, which has been described in the Bible, have been a problem for some people. In the United States it is estimated that 35 million people suffer from all allergies combined, about 9 million of them with asthma. Could it be that the rest of us have developed a tolerance over the ages? It is only an idea.

Where children are concerned, most can eat what they like, play with animals, go everywhere, and touch just about everything without having to worry about getting troublesome allergic symptoms. And of asthmatic children, about half outgrow their disease. As for contact dermatitis, except for poison ivy, this is rare in children.

Glossary

ALLERGEN. A substance, usually a protein in food, pollen, or mold—the cause of an allergy in some people.

ALLERGIST. A doctor who specializes in allergies.

ALLERGY. A state of sensitivity in a person, gotten by exposure to a particular foreign substance, called an allergen.

ANAPHYLACTIC SHOCK. A prompt and very severe reaction to an allergen that may cause death in a sensitized person.

ANTIBODY. A molecule produced in the body that interacts and neutralizes an antigen.

ANTIGEN. Any substance triggering the body to form antibodies.

ANTIHISTAMINE. A drug that relieves allergic symptoms by counteracting histamine released by cells in an allergic person.

ASTHMA. An allergic condition mainly causing repeated attacks of difficult breathing.

BACTERIUM (pl., BACTERIA). A microscopic organism, rod-shaped, spherical, in pairs or chains; some cause disease like diphtheria, scarlet fever, but some live in the intestines of animals and people harmlessly.

BLOOD SERUM. The fluid colorless part of the blood.
BRONCHIOLES. The smallest tubes in the bronchial tree in the lungs; they end in the air sacs. Their walls are made of muscle.
BRONCHUS (pl., BRONCHI). One of two large branches leading from the windpipe; open airways in the lungs.
CONGESTION. An abnormal accumulation of blood in any part of the body, usually in an irritated swollen area.
CONTACT DERMATITIS. An acute allergic inflammation of the skin, caused by handling substances—chemical, animal, or vegetable—to which a delayed sensitivity has been acquired.
DANDER. Small scales from the hair or feathers of animals, which may cause allergy.
DERMATOGRAPHISM. A physical allergy in people with very sensitive skin; you can write their name by *stroking* the skin with your nail.
DIARRHEA. Abnormally frequent and loose bowels.
ECZEMA. In infants, an eruption of the upper layers of the skin, showing redness, blisters, oozing, crusting scales.
FUNGUS. One class of plants without chlorophyl; includes mushrooms, plant rusts, and smuts; and molds.
HIEROGLYPHICS. Picture writing on tablets used by ancient peoples, Greek and others.
HISTAMINE. A toxic substance released during an allergic reaction.
HYDROCORTISONE. A member of the corticosteroid family of drugs; a hormone produced naturally by the outer part (cortex) of the adrenal glands.
HYPERSENSITIVITY. The medical name for oversensitivity as to an allergen.
HYPOSENSITIZATION. The process of slowly desensitizing a

person by injections of gradually increased amounts of the allergen.

IDIOSYNCRASY. An intolerance to a drug or a food not of allergic nature.

IMMUNE. A natural or acquired protection against a particular infection.

IMMUNOGLOBULIN E (IgE). The antibody in allergies; of a class of proteins called immunoglobulins.

INFLAMMATION. An abnormal accumulation of blood usually due to an irritant: a chemical, an infection, or the result of an allergy.

INHALANT. Anything breathed in with the air.

MOLD. Microscopic fungus.

MUCOUS MEMBRANE. The lining of body cavities that produce mucus; for example, the nose.

MUCUS. The slimy secretion from mucous glands in the lining of the nose, mouth, and other body openings.

PASSIVE TRANSFER TEST. Indirect skin test using the serum of the allergic person to test for the allergen in a normal, nonsensitized person.

PERENNIAL ALLERGIC RHINITIS. Inflammation of the mucous membrane of the nose due to a nonseasonal allergy.

POLLEN. The microscopic grains, the male fertilizing cells of flowering plants. Many of the airborne pollen grains are allergens.

POLLINOSIS. A seasonal allergy due to pollens.

POLYPS. A protruding growth from a mucous membrane.

REACTION. The way the body responds to a foreign body or substance in an infection or allergy.

RHINITIS. Inflammation of the mucous membrane of the nose.

SENSITIZATION. The effect of becoming intolerant to an allergenic substance.

SINUS. One of several cavities in the skull bones that drain into the nose.

SPORE. The reproductive part of fungi and other microscopic organisms. The spores of certain molds are allergens.

STAMEN. The male part of a flower that produces pollen.

URTICARIA. Smooth, slightly elevated patches (wheals) of the skin. Also called hives, an allergic reaction.

VIRUS. Tiny forms, not visible with the light microscope; are parasitic: can live only within living cells.

WHEAL. A white bump appearing on the skin in an allergic reaction, as in hives.

Further Reading

Benack, Raymond T. *What Is Allergy: A Guide for the Allergic Person.* Philadelphia: J. B. Lippincott, 1967.

Blaine, Tom R. *Goodbye Allergies.* New York: Citadel Press, 1968.

Forsythe, Elizabeth. *Asthma, Hay Fever and Other Allergies and How to Live with Them.* Levittown, N.Y.: Transatlantic, 1976.

Gerrard, John W. *Understanding Allergies.* Springfield, Ill.: Chas. C. Thomas, 1973.

Joseph, Lou, in consultation with Mills, Alice S. (M.D.). *A Doctor Discusses Allergy Fact and Fallacies.* Chicago, Ill.: Budlong Press, 1975.

Mackarness, Richard. *Eating Dangerously: Hidden Hazards of Food Allergies.* New York: Harcourt Brace Jovanovich, 1976.

Rapaport, Howard G., and Linde, Shirley Motter. *The Complete Allergy Guide.* New York: Simon & Schuster, 1971.

Rapp, Doris J. *Allergies and Your Child.* New York: Holt, Rinehart & Winston, 1972.

PAMPHLETS

For booklets on allergy you can write to the Allergy Foundation of America, 801 Second Avenue, New York, N.Y. 10017 (212) 867-8875.

Hay Fever	50¢
Handbook for the Asthmatic	50¢
Allergy in Children	50¢
The Skin and Its Allergies	50¢
Insect Stings	25¢
Mold Allergy	25¢
Food Allergy	25¢
Drug Allergy	25¢
Cosmetic Allergy	25¢
Asthma, Climate and Weather	25¢
Allergic Diseases	Single Copies Free
Answers to Some Questions About Allergy	Single Copies Free

Index

Adrenalin, 32
Allergen, 2, 4, 6–7
Allergies
    allergens, 2, 4, 6–7
    asthma, 29–34, 54, 55
    chemicals, 7, 51, 53–54
    contact dermatitis, 7, 16, 48–55
    dermatographism, 40
    drug sensitivity, 7, 40, 54
    food, 2, 3, 6–7, 35–38
    hay fever, 24–28
    heredity and, 2, 4, 18, 31
    insect stings, 41–47
    mold, 1, 6, 12, 21–22, 38
    patch test, 16, 53
    rhinitis, 1, 17–23
    skin tests, 13, 15, 21, 23, 37
    transfer test, 15
Allergist, 3, 9
Amino acids, 28
Anaphylactic shock, 42, 54
Animals, 6, 12, 21
Antibodies, 2–4
Antigen, 2
Antihistamines, 23, 44, 50
Asthma, 29–34, 54, 55

Bacterium, 1–2
Blood serum, 15, 27, 54
Breast-feeding, 35
Bronchi, 19, 29
Bronchioles, 29–30, 32

Capillaries, 27
Carbon dioxide, 30
Challenging procedure, 37
Chemicals, 7, 51, 53–54
Colds, 2
Contact dermatitis, 7, 16, 48–55
Corticosteroids, 32, 34
Cortisone, 36
Cromolyn, 34

Dander, 6, 12, 21
Delayed hypersensitivity, 48
Dermatographism, 40
Diagnosis, 16
Diagnostic aids, 26
Diarrhea, 8
Drug sensitivity, 7, 40, 54

Eczema, 31, 35–36
Edema, 27

Emotional stress, 38, 40
Eosinophiles, 19, 30
Epinephrine, 32, 44

Farmers' lung, 12
Food allergy, 2, 3, 6–7, 35–38
Fungus, 1–2

Hay fever, 24–28
Heredity, 2, 4, 18, 31
Hieroglyphics, 41
Histamine, 4, 27, 31, 34, 41, 48
Hives, 36, 38
Hormones, 32
House dust, 21–23
Hydrocortisone, 50
Hypersensitivity, 1
Hyposensitization, 23, 27, 28, 32, 44–45, 47

Idiosyncrasy, 54
Immunity, 3, 35
Immunoglobulin E, (IgE), 27–28, 31
Infection, 1–4, 18, 31
Influenza (flu), 2
Ingestants, 6–7
Inhalants, 6
Injectables, 7
Insect stings, 41–47

Mast cells, 27
Measles, 2, 3
Medicines, 23, 28, 32, 34, 44, 50
Mold allergy, 1, 6, 12, 21–22, 38
Mucous membrane, 18
Mucus, 30, 32
Mumps, 2

Oxygen, 19, 30

Passive transfer test, 15
Patch test, 16, 53
Penicillin, 7, 54
Perennial allergic rhinitis, 1
Pets, 6, 12, 21
Physical examination, 11–12, 18
Poison ivy, 7, 48, 50–51, 55
Pollen, 6, 24–28, 38
Pollen count, 26
Pollinosis, 24–28
Polyps, 21
Protein, 2, 25
Puncture test, 15

Ragweed, 6, 25–26
Reaction, 1
Rhinitis, 1, 17–23
Ringworm, 2

Scarlet fever, 2
Scratch test, 13
Sensitization, 4, 41, 42
Sinuses, 21
Skin tests, 13, 15, 21, 23, 37
Spores, 6, 22
Stamen, 24
Synthetic nonallergenic diet, 38

Target (shock) organs, 8
Transfer test, 15

Urticaria (hives), 36, 38
Urushiol, 51

Virus, 1–2, 31

Wheals, 8, 13
Whooping cough, 2

About the Author

Sarah R. Riedman is the author of over thirty books for young readers, specializing in scientific subjects. She is a physiologist, medical writer, and editor, and has taught college level biology, physiology, and hygiene. Ms. Riedman is a member of the American Association of Medical Writers (Fellow), the New York Academy of Sciences, World Federation of Scientific Workers, and the American Association for Advancement of Science. Sarah R. Riedman is also the author of *Sharks* (An Easy-Read Fact Book) recently published by Franklin Watts. She lives in Jensen Beach, Florida.